The 28 Day Plan

DETOX

Christine Green

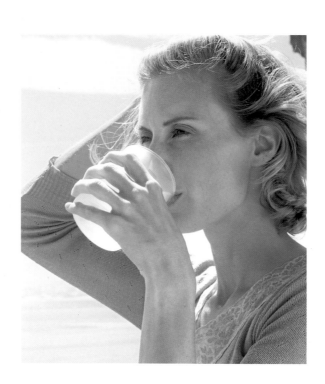

p

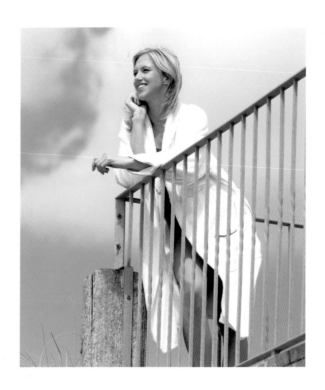

This is a Parragon Publishing Book

This edition published in 2002

Parragon Publishing
Queen Street House
4 Queen Street
Bath BA1 1HE, UK

Copyright © Parragon 2002

Designed, produced and packaged by
Stonecastle Graphics Limited

Text by Christine Green
Edited by Gillian Haslam
Designed by Sue Pressley and Paul Turner
Commissioned photography by Roddy Paine

ISBN 0-75259-354-4

Printed in China

Disclaimer

The exercises and advice detailed in this book
assume that you are a normally healthy adult.
Therefore the author, publishers, their servants, or
agents cannot accept responsibility for loss or
damage suffered by individuals as a result of
following advice or attempting an exercise or
treatment referred to in this book. It is strongly
recommended that individuals intending to
undertake an exercise program and any change of
diet do so following consultation with their medical
practitioner.

Contents

What is Detoxification?

Imagine a well-toned body, the loss of several pounds of weight, healthy skin, increased

energy, better digestion. You feel fit and healthy and able to relax at the drop of a hat –

does it sound too good to be true?

Don't despair – it is possible and it is achievable on a 28-day detox program following which you will feel so much healthier, more energetic, cleansed, and revitalized!

Detoxing is not a diet nor is it a strict eating regime. Just as you would spring-clean your home, when you detox you are in effect spring-cleaning your body, clearing out all the toxins and poisons that have accumulated inside you over the years. Toxins enter the body in many ways – from the air we breathe to the food we eat, from pollutants in the environment to the emotional stresses of everyday life, all these factors can contribute to toxic build-up. After a while they can knock the body off balance, leaving you feeling sluggish and lacking in energy. However, it is possible to eliminate those toxins, to bring the body back into balance, and to return it to good health by detoxing. In doing so you are:

✓ Improving your immune system

✓ Improving your circulation

✓ Ensuring the body has all the necessary energy it requires to "look after and repair" itself

How does it work?

The body is a complex machine and, like any machine, it needs regular maintenance to keep it working efficiently. The body needs a daily intake of fluid and food to provide it with energy, to keep it healthy, and to help repair and renew damaged cells. Food is processed by the body's metabolism. Once the internal

Signs of possible toxic overload
- Allergic reactions
- Bloating and sweating
- Constant tiredness
- Headaches
- Intolerance to fat
- Mood changes
- Poor concentration
- Poor digestion

organs have extracted the nutrients from the foods, the rest is simply waste and is transported to those organs whose role it is to eliminate waste products from the body.

Liver: This organ has many important functions, one of which is to transport unwanted or toxic substances that enter the body and to transform them into substances that the body can either retain or expel.

Kidneys: These filter and eliminate toxins from the blood via the urine. They also ensure that the body has sufficient fluid and that the balance of potassium and sodium, both important elements for regulating the amount of fluids in the body, is maintained.

Lymphatic system: Acting as a waste disposal unit, the lymphatic system is a network of vessels extending all around the body. It produces a liquid called lymph that absorbs micro-organisms, dead cells, excess fluids, and other waste products derived from food. It transports them to the lymph nodes where the fluid is filtered, taken into the bloodstream and on to eliminatory organs where unwanted substances are expelled from the body via urine, faeces, or sweat.

Skin: An important indicator as to what is happening

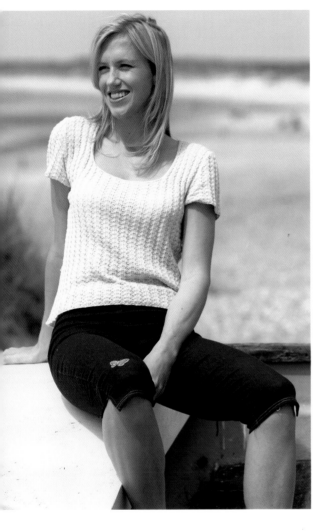

Following the detox program

The greatest attraction about detoxing is the "good-to-be-alive/full-of-energy/I'm raring-to-go" feeling that it produces. Ask anyone who has followed a detox program and they will almost certainly agree that they felt fitter after it than they had done in years. Age is not important – you may be 25 or 55, a full-time housewife or a busy employee climbing up the executive ladder. The simple fact is that we all get stressed, we all rush around too much, and we all tend to eat more convenience food than perhaps we should. Can you imagine how our insides must look? The answer is to detox in order to restore inner cleanliness. The results will be amazing, but you must be determined. You'll need a good helping of willpower to complete the recommended program.

within our body and the overall state of our health. As an organ, it excretes large quantities of waste, such as urea, salts, uric acid, ammonia, and water.

If these organs do not work efficiently, our long-term health will invariably suffer and the body will not be able to repair itself following stress or illness. The organs slow down, and the accumulation of waste and toxins builds up to such an extent that toxic overload becomes almost inevitable. This throws the body out of balance, and the only way to restore balance is by following a detoxification program to cleanse the system.

Healthy Eating

The basic principle of our detox program is to eat three well-chosen meals a day – breakfast, lunch, and dinner – allowing at least five hours between them to allow the body enough time to process the food before the next meal.

If possible, try to eat the last meal of the day no later than 7.00pm; this gives the body ample time to digest the food before you go to bed.

Choosing what to eat is half the fun of the program. While it is very specific in the sense that if foods are not listed, they should not be eaten, there are so many delicious dishes that are recommended that you will be spoiled for choice.

But do not worry if your culinary skills are not quite up to cordon bleu standard, don't worry; it is amazing how different a salad can taste with the addition of some herbs or a few nuts sprinkled over the top.

Fresh fruit and vegetables are a major part of the detox program, largely because of the abundance of minerals and vitamins that they contain. Canned and processed foods are best avoided as they contain additives and preservatives. However, if you do find yourself having to eat some, make sure that most of that meal is salad or lightly steamed vegetables.

Recommended fruit

- Apples
- Apricots
- Bilberries
- Blackberries
- Blackcurrants
- Blueberries
- Cherries
- Cranberries
- Currants
- Damsons
- Dates
- Figs
- Golden sultanas
- Gooseberries
- Grapefruit
- Grapes
- Greengages
- Guavas
- Kiwi fruit
- Lemons
- Limes
- Loganberries
- Lychees
- Mangoes
- Melons
- Mulberries
- Nectarines
- Passionfruit
- Paw-paw
- Peaches
- Pears
- Pineapple
- Plums
- Pomegranates
- Prunes
- Quinces
- Raspberries
- Redcurrants
- Rhubarb
- Strawberries

Recommended vegetables

- Artichokes
- Asparagus
- Beans (broad, butter, French, haricot, mung, red kidney, runner)
- Beansprouts
- Beet
- Broccoli
- Brussels sprouts
- Cabbage (red, savoy, spring, white, winter)
- Carrots
- Cauliflower
- Celeriac
- Celery
- Chicory
- Chinese leaf
- Cucumbers
- Eggplant
- Endive
- Fennel
- Kohlrabi
- Leeks
- Lettuce
- Okra
- Onions
- Parsnips
- Peas
- Peppers (bell, capsicum)
- Plantain
- Potatoes
- Pumpkins
- Radishes
- Scallions
- Spring greens
- Swede
- Sweetcorn
- Sweet potatoes
- Squashes
- Turnips
- Watercress
- Yams
- Zucchini

Recommended nuts

High in calories, nuts are also high in fiber, nutrients, and potassium so are an ideal source of unsaturated fatty acids. Best eaten raw, unsalted, and fresh. Choose from the following:

- Almonds
- Brazils
- Cashews
- Chestnuts
- Hazelnuts
- Macadamia
- Pecans
- Pine nuts
- Pistachios
- Walnuts

Recommended seeds, pulses, and herbs

Just as nuts are high in nutrients, so too are pulses and seeds. Once fully sprouted, their nutrient content becomes higher. Great for adding flavor and color to foods.

Pulses and seeds:
- Alfalfa
- Cardamom pods
- Chickpeas
- Chilies
- Pumpkin seeds
- Sesame seeds
- Sunflower seeds

Herbs:
- Cayenne pepper
- Basil
- Cilantro
- Dill
- Fennel
- Ginger
- Lemon grass
- Marjoram
- Parsley
- Pepper
- Rosemary
- Sage
- Tarragon
- Thyme

Recommended fish

Fish is a perfect food as it contains all the vital proteins. As with most food, it is healthier if eaten fresh rather than frozen; freezing depletes fish of many of its essential nutrients. Smoked fish is fine provided it has been treated naturally. Avoid eating fish in brine – it is too salty. If selecting canned fish, those preserved in olive or vegetable oil are the best.

- Cod
- Crab
- Haddock
- Halibut
- Herring
- Lemon sole
- Lobster
- Mackerel
- Monkfish
- Pilchards
- Plaice
- Salmon
- Sardines
- Shrimp
- Skate
- Trout
- Tuna

Foods to avoid

- Artificial sweeteners
- Avocados
- Bananas
- Bread
- Cow's milk/cheese
- Food additives or preservatives
- Lentils
- Mushrooms
- Oranges
- Red meat
- Salt
- Spinach
- Sugar
- Tomatoes

Other recommended foods

Other foods that are important in your detox program and that can help to add flavor to meals include:

- Balsamic vinegar
- Cider vinegar
- Grapeseed oil
- Miso mustard
- Olive oil
- Olives
- Quorn
- Rice cakes
- Seaweed
- Sesame oil
- Tahini
- Tofu
- Walnut oil

If you cannot find them in your supermarket, then most health food stores will stock them.

Recommended non-dairy products

- Goat's milk/cheese/yogurt
- Sheep's milk/cheese/yogurt
- Rice milk
- Soya milk

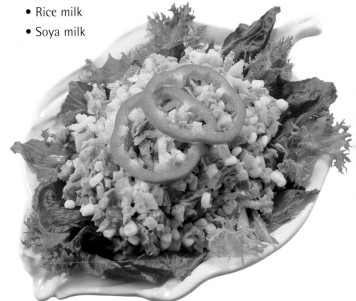

Healthy Drinking

Maintaining a healthy balance of fluids is always essential, especially when you consider that the body is made up of 80 per cent water, but when detoxing it is particularly important to increase your intake of fluid to help cleanse the system and flush out any impurities.

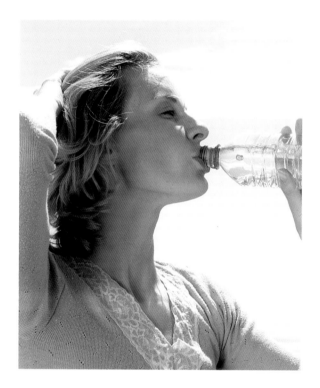

Fruit juices: These can be drunk in addition to the recommended quantity of water. If buying pre-packed, check the label that it is pure, unsweetened juice and not the variety made up in water from fruit pulp. Better still, if you have a juicer make your own.

Apple juice
2 medium-sized hard apples

There is no need to peel the apple, simply chop it up roughly and pop the pieces into the juicer. Rich in vitamin C, this is an excellent liver and kidney cleanser and assists the growth and development of a healthy nervous system.

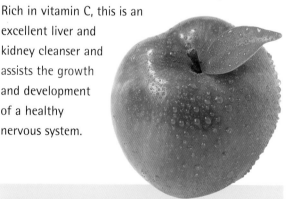

Water: Your aim must be to drink at least 3 pints of water a day. That may seem a lot and likely to cause several unscheduled visits to the loo, but after several days the body will adjust. And if drinking plain water becomes a little boring, try adding lemon, lime, honey, or ginger to flavor it.

Herbal teas: Echinacea and fenugreek are reputedly the best.

Dandelion coffee: Available from health food shops, this is sometimes drunk as an alternative to coffee.

Home-made fruit juices to try
If you have a juicer, you can make your own fresh juice using any of the following fruits:

- Apples
- Grapes
- Grapefruit
- Lemons
- Limes
- Mango
- Melons
- Papaya
- Peaches
- Pears
- Pineapple
- Strawberries
- Watermelon

Grapefruit juice
1¹/₂ grapefruits

The pink ones are great for this as they are slightly sweeter than other types. Peel off the skin but leave on the pith. Chop up the fruit roughly and then put the pieces into the juicer. Grapefruit contains pectin which can help to lower blood cholesterol and half a grapefruit provides more than half the daily requirement of vitamin C.

Peach juice
2 medium-sized peaches

Leave the skin on, cut the fruit in half, remove the stone, and then put it into the juicer. Peach juice is ideal for helping to cleanse the intestines and colon. It also helps to regulate blood fat levels, maintains healthy skin and assists in the healing of wounds.

Home-made vegetable juices
Some vegetables can also be juiced successfully. The choice is varied, but beet, carrot, celery, cucumber, and watercress all make delicious drinks and are full of vitamins.

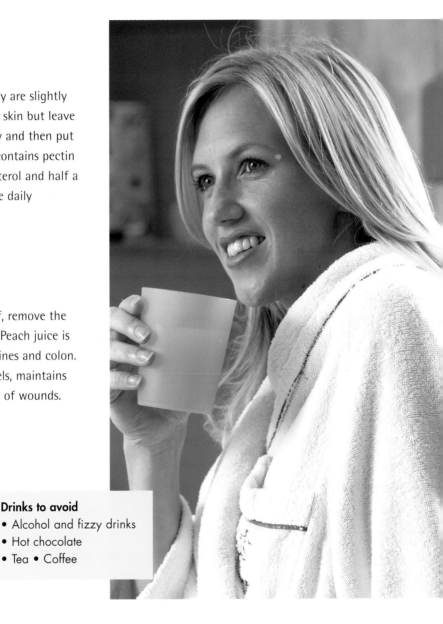

Drinks to avoid
- Alcohol and fizzy drinks
- Hot chocolate
- Tea • Coffee

Carrot juice
3 large carrots

With a slightly spicy taste, carrot juice can be made extra tasty by adding some freshly chopped herbs. Simply wash and slice the carrots, and pop them into the juicer. Carrot juice is a very good source of fiber and helps to boost immunity. It helps to cleanse the liver of excess fats, aids digestion, and is an excellent source of vitamin A.

Beet juice
¹/₃ medium-sized beet

Raw beet is better than cooked beetroot. Wash it thoroughly and remove any roots. Then slice it and put the pieces into the juicer. Beet juice is excellent for cleansing the blood and kidneys and aids the development of a healthy nervous system.

Planning What You Can Eat

By changing your eating habits and eating healthy foods regularly, your energy levels will be maintained throughout the day, you will feel more alert, and you will not be piling on extra pounds with that mid-morning chocolate bar.

The detox program is not a diet and so you should serve yourself adequate helpings that each day should include:

- Three portions of vegetables
- Three portions of fruit
- Three portions of salad
- One portion of non-dairy yogurt, cheese, or milk
- Two portions of nuts or fish
- One portion of brown rice

The above list may seem a little daunting to you, especially if you generally skip breakfast, grab a quick sandwich for lunch, and perhaps rustle up a shepherd's pie for supper.

The best advice when it comes to planning your daily eating schedule is to draw up some menus a week in advance so that you will know what you are eating for breakfast, lunch, and dinner on each of the days ahead.

Methods of cooking

If cooking is not your forte, then you will love the detox program because there is practically no cooking involved! In general, the less food is heated, the more nutrients it will retain. Of course, there are exceptions, such as fish which must be thoroughly cooked. If you prefer your vegetables slightly cooked, then avoid

boiling, slow-cooking, or frying them; use other methods, such as stir frying, broiling, or just pop them into the microwave – these are far tastier and less likely to impair the natural flavor and nutrients in the food.

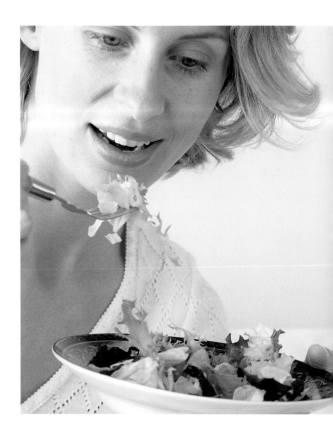

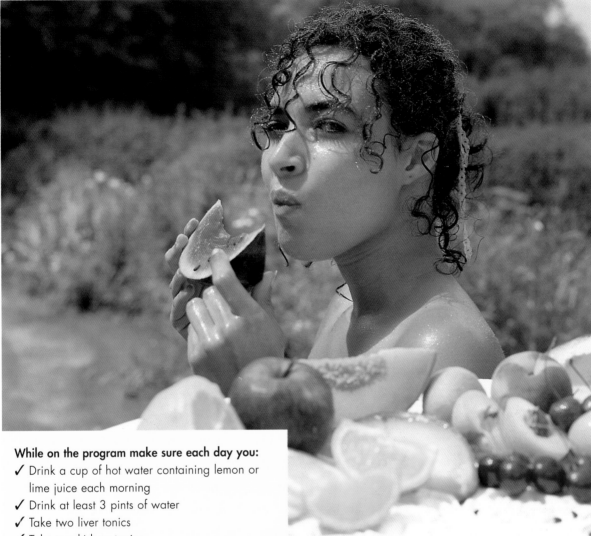

While on the program make sure each day you:
- ✓ Drink a cup of hot water containing lemon or lime juice each morning
- ✓ Drink at least 3 pints of water
- ✓ Take two liver tonics
- ✓ Take two kidney tonics
- ✓ Take a kelp supplement
- ✓ Take a multivitamin supplement for the first 15 days
- ✓ Eat three meals a day
- ✓ Eat one portion of rice (preferably brown short grain)
- ✓ Eat three portions of vegetables (one of which should be raw)
- ✓ Eat three portions of fruit
- ✓ Eat three portions of fresh salad
- ✓ Eat one portion of a non-dairy product

Calorie intake

All foods contain calories which are a measure of the amount of energy contained in that particular food. The number of calories your body requires each day largely depends on your age, lifestyle, etc. The general consensus is that the average woman needs approximately 1600 calories per day. If the calorie intake is reduced to lower than 1000, then the body is not getting enough to function properly and will begin to go into starvation mode.

Daily Treatments

To achieve the goal of the detox program – a cleansed inner body and an invigorated spirit – it is important that you follow the recommendations on page 11 throughout your 28-day plan.

Why certain foods are important

Hot lemon water: Starting the day with a cup of hot water and a squeeze of lemon or lime juice will freshen your mouth and give a kick-start to your liver (the largest organ involved in detoxing).

Water: Cleansing, restoring, and rejuvenating the body are the three basic principles of a detox program and the one vital ingredient which can help is water. So make sure you drink plenty of it.

Liver tonic: The liver should be treated with kid gloves throughout the 28-day program so that it does its job of detoxification efficiently. To help do this, it needs a tonic in the shape of at least two of the following foods each day:

- Two cups of fennel or dandelion tea
- A medium-sized glass of pure carrot or beet juice
- Eat a medium-sized bunch of grapes
- Include a fresh clove of garlic in your food

Kidney tonic: Like the liver, the kidneys have a hard job to do in detoxing the system. Including certain foods in your diet will enable them to work more efficiently. Each day follow two of these suggestions:

- Sip a teaspoon of fresh honey dissolved in a cup of hot water
- Drink a medium-sized glass of freshly squeezed cranberry juice
- Eat half a medium-sized melon

Supplements: When you change your eating habits significantly, your metabolic rate is often affected; if sufficient quantities of foods are not consumed, the body begins slowing down. At the start of your program, you may find it helpful to take certain supplements, such as kelp which equips the body with enough iodine to balance the metabolism.

Vitamin supplements: It is often a good idea to include an all-round vitamin supplement in the initial stages of your detox program to ensure that the body is not being depleted of any essential nutrients. Generally the body adjusts after two weeks of the program and you can stop taking the supplements.

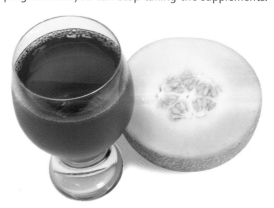

Each day throughout your detox program:

✓ Take a cold shower/bath
✓ Do some self-massage
✓ Perform 30 minutes of exercises
✓ Spend five minutes on quality breathing
✓ Spend ten minutes enjoying some relaxation
✓ Do five minutes of visualization exercises
✓ Smile or laugh heartily every day
✓ Exfoliate every three days
✓ Take an Epsom salts bath every five days

T.L.C. (Tender Loving Care)

The detox program can only really be hailed as a success if the entire "person", inside and outside, has been cleansed and restored. This is where a combination of exercise, relaxation and pampering comes in.

The benefits of a cold shower

Refreshing, invigorating and rejuvenating, a morning shower is just what the body needs to jump-start it into action. But when you are nearly finished, gradually turn on the cold faucet allowing cold water to run over your body for one minute. This might sound uncomfortable but that minute of cold water will:

✓ tone up the skin
✓ tone up the muscles
✓ give the lymphatic system a jump-start

If you don't have a shower, then simply take a bath as usual and, as the water drains away, turn the cold water on, gather it in your cupped hands and splash it over your body. Better still, if you have a shower attachment that you can fit over the cold water faucet, use this to spray yourself with cold water.

Self-massage

There is nothing quite like a full body massage to relieve tension, lower blood pressure and stress levels, eliminate excess fluids and toxins, and give the skin an overall healthy glow. It can be expensive going to a beauty salon, so why not bring the beauty salon to your home and do it yourself? If you have a willing partner to help you, so much the better, otherwise try giving yourself this very simple head massage, ideal for dealing with a tension headache. A five-minute massage will leave you feeling totally relaxed.

1. Begin by taking several deep breaths.
2. Using the thumb and forefinger of each hand, very gently pinch your earlobes and massage the edges of the ears moving all the way round up to the top and pulling them slightly away from the head.
3. Now move on to massage the temples using the first two fingers of each hand.
4. Finally concentrate on the top of the head and apply firm pressure all over the scalp, almost as if you were washing your hair.

Skin brushing

No-one had ever heard of dry skin brushing a few years ago, but now it is one of the "in things" to do. It helps to clean the skin of all the dead cells that clog up the pores, leaving the skin soft and smooth. But that's not all it does. A gentle five-minute daily skin brush is an effective, simple way to boost the lymphatic system. It is also excellent for helping to eliminate most women's number one enemy – cellulite!

How to skin brush

• Take a natural bristle brush or a dry face cloth, begin at the feet and, using small circular strokes, gradually move up the body always brushing toward the heart with gentle, long, and firm movements.
• Never brush away from the heart, this may cause faintness or unsettle the natural flow of the blood.
• Keep each stroke firm as you work your way gradually up the body from the ankles to the knees, from the knees to the top of your thighs and over your buttocks.
• Starting at the wrists, move up the arms to the shoulders and down from the tops of the arms over the shoulders, then gently up the neck to the base of the skull.
• Work over the stomach using gentle strokes in a clockwise direction to prevent upsetting the digestive flow in your intestines. Be extra gentle on the breasts and avoid brushing over the nipples.
• Don't expect to notice changes after the first treatment but once you have done it several times, your skin will begin to feel softer and smoother.

Exercise and Relaxation

Exercise is the ideal way to get the body system going and to increase the metabolic rate.

Some exercises are better suited to the detox program than others.

Walking

Gentle and easy, walking stimulates the heart, lungs, muscles and mind. Begin with 10-15 minutes each day, gradually building up to 30 minutes. Walk fast enough to work up a slight sweat.

Swimming

Swimming works most of the major muscle groups and is an excellent aerobic exercise. Check if there are any classes at your local pool.

Cycling

This is one of the best types of exercise for building muscular endurance and toning up leg muscles. If you don't own a real bike, the same benefits can be derived from an exercise bike – a good reason to join a local gym!

If you haven't exercised for a while:
- Don't exercise too strenuously to begin with – overtired muscles create waste products and put a strain on the lymphatic system
- Whatever exercise you decide to do, begin slowly and then build up gradually
- Don't push yourself too hard
- Try to find an exercise that frees the mind
- Don't choose something you don't like – remember exercise should be enjoyable

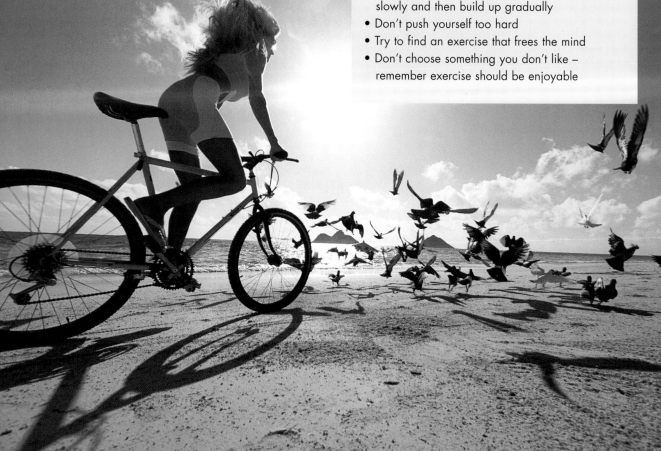

Bouncing

Bouncing on a "mini trampoline" for 5-15 minutes daily is perfect for helping to drain the lymphatic system.

Housework

It's official – a vigorous burst of housework can be as good for you as a trip to the gym, and scrubbing the floor burns up 400 calories an hour! So if you are concerned that your house is getting neglected while you are on the program, you could always integrate housework as one form of exercise. The secret is to do a job in half the time you would normally take, putting the maximum amount of effort in!

Exercise is good for you and it should also be fun. Set some time aside to enjoy an invigorating bike ride or play some favorite music and bounce on a mini trampoline in time with the rhythm.

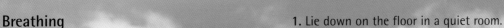

Breathing

Another important element in your detox program is to spend at least five minutes each day on quality deep breathing. Very few of us breathe correctly and whenever we feel tense or worried, our breathing pattern becomes shallow and chest movements erratic. Correct breathing will rectify this. This is the art of deep breathing:

Why learning to breathe correctly is important:
- It helps to cleanse the body
- It teaches you how to relax
- It energizes your body

1. Lie down on the floor in a quiet room.
2. Place both hands on your abdomen, fingertips gently touching.
3. Slowly begin to breathe in through your nose to the count of four.
4. Hold for a few seconds and then, as you exhale to the count of eight, become aware of your stomach expanding and your fingertips parting.
5. Practice this sequence several times.
To begin with it will feel rather strange but persevere and soon you will begin to feel more relaxed and there will be no need to use your fingers to check that your abdomen (rather than your chest) is expanding.

Relaxation

Breathing correctly acts as a natural tranquillizer for the nervous system and so the deeper you breathe, the calmer the mind becomes. Acquiring the ability to relax totally is something very few people achieve but the benefits of practicing relaxation techniques can stand you in good stead for coping with most of life's day-to-day stresses.

Standing in a supermarket queue or waiting in a traffic queue will not seem so irritating once you have learned some simple relaxation exercises. That's not to say you won't have the odd lapse now and again nor that you will always feel calm and together, but it will at least demonstrate that a relaxed state of mind is achievable with a little practice.

Follow these simple steps and don't be surprised if you end up falling asleep!

1. Lie down on a comfortable mat in a quiet room, legs outstretched, arms resting gently by your sides.
2. Close your eyes and take a few slow, deep breaths.
3. As you inhale, tense all the muscles in your body, feel them tighten and become taut. Then, as you exhale, become aware of all the tension ebbing away.
4. Bring your shoulders up to your ears as far as you can, making sure that your head stays flat on the mat, count to five and then slowly drop your shoulders back to their original position.
5. Now for your arms. Tense them; as you do so they will automatically draw in nearer to your body, hold for a count of five, and then release. Become aware of the tension ebbing away as your arms fall limply to either side of your body.
6. Then repeat the tension and relaxation sequence with your abdomen, buttocks, legs, and feet.

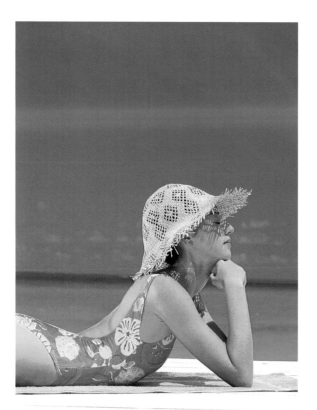

Visualization

Five minutes spent totally submerged in a pleasant make-believe world can be five of the most valuable minutes in your detox program. It is all a matter of concentration.

The objective is to sit back, close your eyes and imagine yourself in any situation which makes you feel happy: lying on a warm beach with the sun beating down, sitting in a field on a bright summer's day, take whatever mental image is a good, positive one for you. Linger over as many details as you are can so making the image come alive. Then, as often as possible, bring this picture to the forefront of your mind keeping the thoughts that are associated with the picture positive and full of energy.

These images or visualizations are ways of helping to see yourself attaining goals and achieving success. When you have been practicing them for a while, you will start to gain confidence and think more positively about yourself.

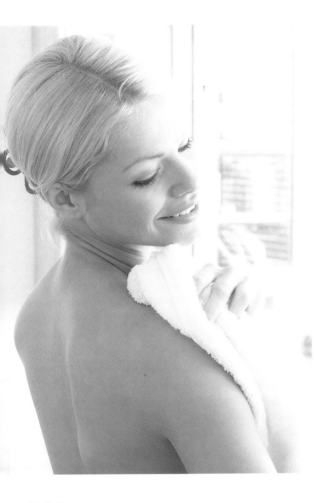

climb back into the bath and carry on rubbing until all the cream has been washed off.

4. Get out of the bath and towel yourself dry before applying moisturizer all over your body.

5. Finally jump into a pair of your warmest pyjamas, and hop into bed with a good book for a restorative early night.

Epsom salts baths

Speed up the elimination of toxins from the skin and improve your circulation with an Epsom salts bath. Run the bath water and add $1/2$-1lb of Epsom salts to the water. Most pharmacies and health food stores sell Epsom salts.

Soak for about 20 minutes, and when you get out, keep yourself warm by piling on lots clothes; this will help the body to continue sweating out toxins.

Exfoliate

Every day exfoliate the skin. Not unlike dry skin brushing, exfoliation clears the skin of dead cells; the main difference is that it needs to be done with water and an exfoliater, so this treatment could easily be integrated with one of your pampering sessions.

1. As you run a bath, add a few drops of your favorite bath oil and relax for at least ten minutes in the water, allowing time for your skin to soften before you begin to exfoliate.

2. You can either apply exfoliation cream while in the bath, lifting each limb out of the water to do so, or climb out of the bath and apply the cream using firm circular movements all over your body. When finished,

Laughter

Can you remember the last time you had a jolly good laugh or was it so long ago, you've forgotten?

Experts have found that people who use humor to cope with stress experience:

✓ Less tension
✓ Less fatigue
✓ Less anger
✓ Less depression

And, furthermore, laughing:

✓ Relaxes face muscles
✓ Exercises internal muscles
✓ Deepens breathing
✓ Improves blood circulation
✓ Lowers blood pressure and releases endorphins, the feel-good chemicals that are the body's natural painkillers

So hire a comedy video, read a funny book, or watch your favorite TV sitcom and have a good laugh.

Good Food

The great thing about the detox program is that it gives you the opportunity to have fun and experiment with a range of different foods.

Use your imagination and create some dishes that may well become a staple part of your diet long after the program has ended. If you are looking for some ideas, here are a few to tempt you.

Breakfast recipes

It's essential to have breakfast and here are some tasty recipes which are quick and easy to prepare.

Pear delight

1 glass apple juice
1 pear
5fl oz goat's or sheep's milk yogurt

Peel the pear and place it in a pan with the apple juice and some water. Bring to the boil and simmer until the pear has softened. Place the pear in a breakfast bowl and pour the yogurt over it.

Muesli

Oats
Golden raisins
Sesame seeds
Hazelnuts
Sunflower seeds
Sheep's milk yogurt

Simply mix two dessertspoons of each dry ingredient in a bowl and soak them overnight in enough water to make the mixture slightly moist. In the morning serve with sheep's milk yogurt.

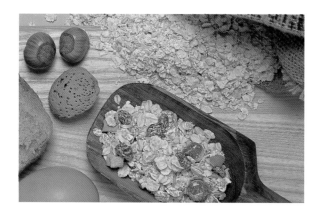

Porridge

Jumbo porridge oats
Water
Handful of golden raisins

Put the oats into the bowl and stir in some water to the desired consistency. Then add a handful of raisins for sweetness.

Oats

Raw oats
$1/2$ chopped apple
1-2 tablespoons golden raisins
$1/2$ teaspoon cinnamon
Tablespoon raw honey

Put quarter of a cup of raw unprocessed oats in a dish with some distilled water and leave overnight to soak. The next morning add the remaining ingredients, stir and enjoy.

Lunchtime recipes

These suggestions are quick to prepare, and provide something light but nutritious and healthy to keep you going until your evening meal.

Potato salad

Portion cooked new potatoes
1 red onion, chopped
Lemon juice
Olive oil
1 tablespoon pine nuts
Portion cooked shrimp
1 fennel bulb, chopped

Cook the new potatoes in a pan of boiling water. When almost cooked, drain and slice each in half. Fry the chopped onion and fennel in the olive oil until translucent. Add the potato halves and fry until everything is slightly browned. While browning the vegetables, lightly toast the pine nuts. When the vegetables are almost done, add the shrimp and pine nuts, cook for a further 2 minutes. Toss the whole salad together and dress with a drizzle of fresh lemon juice.

Rice salad

$1/2$ green bell pepper, deseeded and cored
$1/2$ red bell pepper, deseeded and cored
2in piece of cucumber
$1/4$ cup boiled brown rice, rinsed and drained
$1/4$ cup cooked peas
$1/4$ cup cooked sweetcorn
Soy sauce
Black pepper
Pinch of salt

Chop the peppers and cucumber very finely and mix in with the rice, peas, and sweetcorn. Add the soy sauce and season to taste.

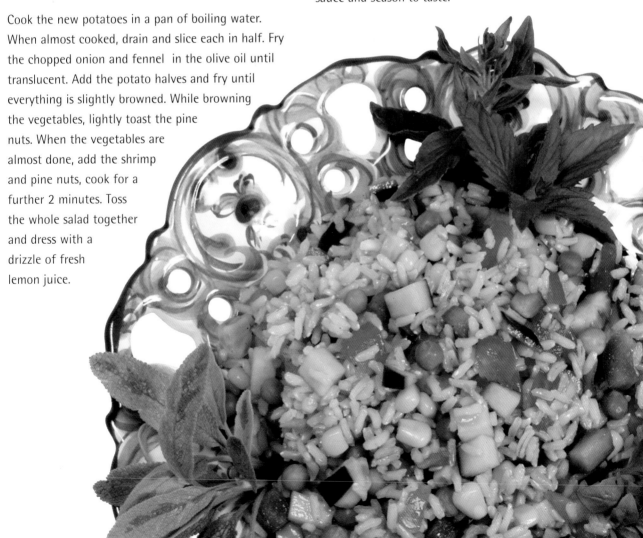

Jacket potato

1 large potato
Olive oil
Portion fresh tuna
2 small chicory bulbs
Balsamic vinegar

Bake the potato until soft. Pre-heat the broiler. Drizzle a little olive oil over a piece of fresh tuna and broil until it begins to turn light brown. Slice the chicory, place strips on top of the tuna and brown under the broiler for the last few minutes. Make a dressing from two teaspoons of olive oil and some balsamic vinegar to taste. Serve the tuna with the jacket potato, pouring the dressing over the fish.

Watercress soup

Enough for two or three servings.
$1^1/_2$ pints vegetable stock
1 large onion, finely chopped
1 clove garlic, crushed
1 lb potatoes, scrubbed and cubed
Large pinch mixed dried herbs
Sea salt
Freshly ground black pepper
Bunch watercress, washed and chopped

Heat 3-4 tablespoons of the vegetable stock in a large saucepan. Add the onion, garlic, and potatoes. Cook on a medium heat for 5 minutes, then bring to the boil. Add the herbs, salt, and pepper and cook until potatoes are tender (approximately 20 minutes). Add the watercress and cook for a further 5 minutes. Cool slightly, then pour into the liquidizer and blend until smooth. Return to the saucepan, reheat gently, stirring in more of the remaining stock or adding water if the soup is still too thick.

Bean salad

Full of protein and a satisfying lunch to keep those hunger pangs at bay. This recipe makes enough for a family of four.
7oz can red kidney beans
7oz can cut green beans
7oz can chickpeas
7oz can butter beans
1 red onion, chopped
1 red pepper, deseeded and chopped
3 stalks celery, finely sliced
$^1/_2$ cup golden raisins
5fl oz sheep's yogurt
Salt and pepper

Drain the beans and chickpeas and place in a large bowl. Add the onion, pepper, celery, and golden raisins, stir in the yogurt, and season to taste. If you wish, this can be served with a green salad.

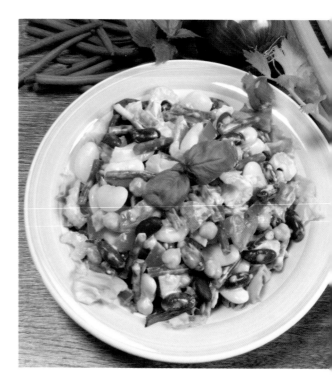

Dinner recipes

The following dishes are perfect either for entertaining guests or to eat as your main meal of the day.

Cod and potato

1 cod steak
2 large potatoes
1 small leek, shredded
1 piece of green cabbage, shredded
1 clove garlic, crushed
Olive oil
Freshly ground black pepper

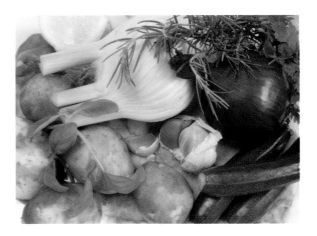

Peel, chop, and boil the potatoes until they are soft. Place the cod under the broiler and cook on both sides until slightly golden. Put a small amount of olive oil into a pan and fry the shredded leek, cabbage, and garlic until slightly browned. Add a tablespoonful of olive oil to the potatoes and mash until creamy. Place the mashed potato in the center of a plate, put the grilled cod on top, and season with black pepper.

Savory potatoes

This dish is savory, tasty, and delicious.
5–6 medium-sized new potatoes
Olive oil
1 small onion, sliced
1 small fennel bulb, sliced
1-2 sprigs of rosemary
2 cloves garlic, crushed
1 small zucchini, sliced
1 tablespoon lemon juice
Fresh basil and cilantro, chopped

Boil the new potatoes until soft. Heat three tablespoons of olive oil in a skillet and fry the onion, fennel, and rosemary until they are soft and lightly browned. Drain the potatoes and add them to the skillet. Add the garlic and zucchini and fry for 10 minutes until the potatoes are browned. Remove from the heat, add the lemon juice, basil, and cilantro, remove the rosemary and serve.

Vegetable bake

3 medium onions, chopped
3-4 carrots, diced
2 large potatoes, peeled and sliced
10fl oz vegetable stock
2 teaspoons dried mint
1 tablespoon olive oil
2 cloves garlic, crushed
Sea salt
Freshly ground black pepper
1 tablespoon sesame seeds

Preheat the oven to 400°F/200°C. Place the onions, carrots and potatoes in a saucepan with the vegetable stock. Bring to the boil then simmer for about 15 minutes. Lightly oil a casserole dish and pour the onions, carrots, and stock from the saucepan in it, plus the mint and seasoning. Layer the sliced potatoes over the top with garlic and sesame seeds sprinkled over and pop in the oven for approximately 30 minutes or until the potatoes turn golden brown.

Delicious desserts

Apple surprise
1 large eating apple
Mixture of cherries, raspberries, strawberries
1 tablespoon honey, plus 1 extra teaspoon
1 tablespoon sheep's milk yogurt
Sesame seeds, toasted

Peel and core the apple, place it in a pan with a small
amount of water and steam gently until the fruit is
tender. In a separate pan, simmer the soft fruits with
the honey until they are soft. Place the apple
on a plate, top with the summer fruits,
and pour the honey and juice over.
Top with a tablespoonful of yogurt
mixed with a teaspoon of honey
and sprinkle with sesame seeds.

Fruit ice
Handful each of raspberries, blackcurrants
and strawberries
1 tablespoon honey
1 small pot of sheep's yogurt

Remove stalks from the fruit and simmer very gently
in a saucepan with the honey until soft. Transfer the
mixture to a bowl and leave to cool. When cool, put
the bowl into the freezer. Keep checking and just
before it is almost frozen, remove from the freezer.
Pour the yogurt into a blender and gradually spoon in
the fruit. Blend in short bursts as the mixture is
added. Serve straight away or
return to the freezer
for a short while.

Strawberry delight
2 small pots goat's milk yogurt
10 large strawberries

Hull the strawberries and put them
in a blender. Add the yogurt and
blend into a delicious
smoothy. Easy!

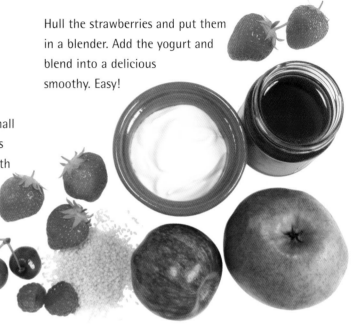

Safe snacking
One of the biggest problems when following any new
diet is that you have to change eating habits. Whereas
you may normally grab a quick sandwich at lunchtime
or meet up with friends for a coffee and a cake, you
now have to be prepared to do things differently.

The one thing to remember on the detox program
is not to skip meals. Be prepared. If you are going out,
for instance take along some of your own snack
foods, a bag of dried fruit, or a rice cake. If you find
that you are peckish midway through the afternoon
and are tempted to raid the cookie jar, don't. Have a
piece of fresh fruit instead or make yourself a cup of
herbal tea.

Work: Most businesses and offices with canteen
facilities cater for a wide variety of diets, so you
should find something to suit you. Alternatively, you
can take something with you and ask a member of

the canteen staff to pop it in the microwave at lunchtime.

Shopping: If you have arranged to meet up with friends in town, there are plenty of places where you can enjoy a jacket potato or a light salad. You could ask for a glass of hot water or herbal tea to drink.

Dining out: There may well be occasions when you are on your detox program when you want to go out for a meal with friends. Whether you are dining in a high-class restaurant or a corner bistro, most establishments are only too willing to accommodate special requests and make up some alternative dishes.

And if you are eating in a Chinese or Indian restaurant where vegetable dishes tend to be highly spiced, select a suitable main dish and perhaps ask for a portion of plain boiled rice. Never be afraid to ask.

Snacks

Although you should never feel really hungry while on the detox program, there are bound to be days when you do feel peckish. Don't be tempted to dive into the cookie jar – there are lots of other alternatives from which you can choose:

✓ Rice cakes (non-salted)
✓ Piece of fresh fruit
✓ Handful of nuts and seeds
✓ Hummus

Remember while on the detox program:
- Never miss a meal
- If you are out, be prepared and take along something to eat, perhaps dried fruit and nuts stored in a plastic bag
- Remember to tell your friends that you are on a detox program
- If dining out, don't be afraid to ask the kitchen staff to make you up a salad

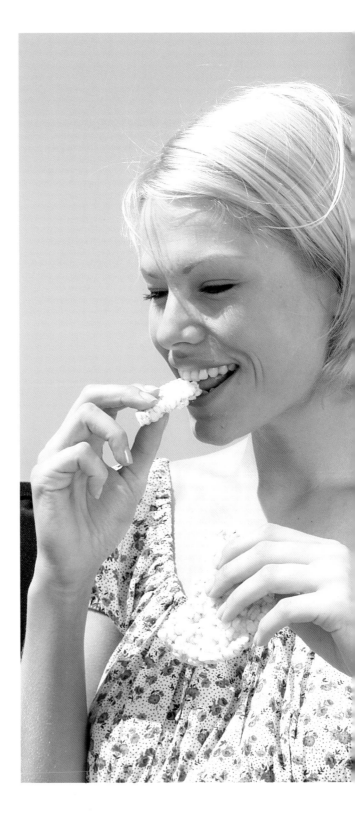

Maintaining The Detox

There are bound to be times during the 28-day detox program when you will feel like giving it all up. These negative thoughts are only to be expected; ignore them, after all they are only thoughts.

To buck yourself up, consider adding some extra rewards into your program. You might treat yourself to a pedicure, take yourself off to the shops and buy yourself a small gift, write yourself a letter of encouragement and put it in the back of your diary to read when the program is over, or relax and listen to some favorite music.

Why not take an aromatherapy bath adding some drops of essential oils to the water that will help boost the elimination of toxins and make you feel relaxed? Six drops of your favorite oil are all you need, and a 20-minute soak will rejuvenate and energize you.

Facial scrub

To clear your complexion, improve the circulation, and tone up slack muscles, try giving yourself a gentle facial scrub. Apply it with small circular movements over the face and neck before rinsing off with warm water.

Facial scrub for dry skin: Blend one tablespoon of ground almonds with clear honey to form a paste. Apply it over the face and then rinse off with tepid water.

Facial scrub for normal skin: Mix one tablespoon of wheatgerm and one tablespoon of light cream together in a basin until they form a paste. Then massage it gently over the skin and rinse away with tepid water.

Relaxing oils
camomile • lavender • sandalwood • ylang ylang
Revitalizing oils
geranium • grapefruit • lemon • lime
Soothing oils
juniper • lavender • marjoram • rosemary

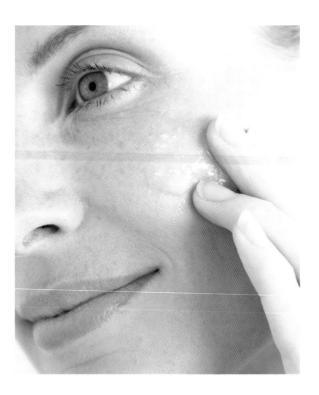

Facial scrub for oily skin: Add one tablespoon of sugar to the soap lather and apply it when washing the face. Rinse with tepid water.

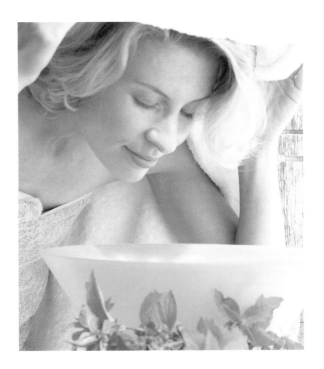

Facial sauna

A facial sauna is a wonderful way to cleanse and relax the skin, encourage the release of nutrients, and eliminate toxins from your skin. For an extra treat add some of your favorite herbs.

1. Remove any make-up and tie your hair back.
2. Boil a pan of water and pour it into a heatproof bowl. If you wish, at this point you can add a handful of your favorite herbs to the water.
3. With a towel draped over your head, lean forward over the bowl, allowing the hot steam to rise and cleanse your face.
4. Remain in the same position for 15 minutes to allow enough time for the pores to open.

After the steam sauna, don't rub or massage your skin. Leave it to dry of its own accord before applying a facemask. If you have thin blood vessels or severe skin blemishes and want to use a facemask to get rid of them, don't use a facial sauna first because it will aggravate the problem.

Some herbs to add to your facial sauna:
Camomile – soothing and cool
Fennel – stimulating and soothing
Geranium – healing and rejuvenating
Lavender – the flowers and leaves are antiseptic
Lemon balm – soothing and astringent

Health problems

It is worth pointing out that you may experience a few health problems while the body is detoxing. Don't worry – this is just nature's way of cleansing the body and ridding it of toxins. They generally clear up by themselves but if symptoms persist or you really don't feel well, then see your doctor. Don't ignore what your body is telling you. Some of the more common problems are:

Constipation: A change in diet nearly always has some effect on the bowels; it should not persist for more than a couple of days. Stools may also be looser than usual due to an increased intake of fiber.

Flu symptoms: Possibly the result of the change in diet. If they are still apparent ten days into the program, check what you are eating and make sure that you are not overdoing exercise.

Fuzzy tongue: Demonstrating that the body is eliminating toxins.

Headache: The result of caffeine and other chemicals being eliminated from the body.

Spots: The skin is the body's biggest organ of elimination and so spots are very common during a detox program.

Tiredness: The first few days will be hard as the body adjusts to your new diet. As you persevere, you will begin to feel more energetic. If your energy levels continue to seem depleted, you may not be eating enough.

Detox Days 1–7

Right, the time has come! You've made all your preparations, and you know what the next 28 days hold. The best and most effective way of undertaking the program is to start on a positive note.

It is good to begin on a Friday as this gives you the weekend to establish a routine. Whether you are a working woman or a busy mother at home, the next 28 days may witness the biggest changes you are ever going to make in your life, so be prepared. Fill in a chart to record each day – you could photocopy the example on page 31 and stick it on your kitchen wall so that you will remember what you must do on each day of the program.

It's important to keep a diary in which you can record your day's activities, what you ate, how you took time out for yourself, and then at the end of

each day make a note of how you felt. Obviously on some days you will find more to write about than others, but by keeping a diary and referring to it when you have negative days, you will keep yourself motivated. You may also wish to keep a record of your weight and measurements using the simple chart on the next page.

Here is a typical plan for the first day but naturally times and the order in which activities are done may differ according to your own lifestyle and some daytime activities can be carried out in the evening when work commitments are over.

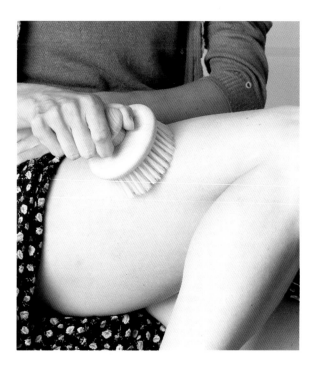

7.00am Drink a glass of hot water with a squeeze of fresh lemon or lime juice in it when you wake up. This will give the body a kick-start.
Invigorate the skin with a dry skin brush followed by a shower or bath. Massage the skin.
8.00am Time for breakfast. Try muesli made from sheep's milk yogurt, sunflower, sesame and pumpkin seeds with chopped dried apricots. Mix the seeds and apricots together and sprinkle over the top of a bowl of yogurt.
9.00am Give yourself a facial.
11.00am Time for relaxation and quality breathing.
1.00pm Lunch. Why not try a salad today and choose from the selection of recipes on pages 18-19? Finish with a piece of fruit. Make sure you eat your meal slowly and give your food time to digest before leaving the table.

2.00pm Relax for a while, read a book or watch the TV. Then go out for a brisk walk, starting off at a slow pace, then speeding up before gradually slowing down again. Plan your route so that it will take you at least 35 minutes to complete.

4.00pm Time for some pampering before you prepare the evening meal. Perhaps give yourself a foot massage – you might well need it after the walk. Place both hands flat on the tops of your feet, then brush them up toward your knees in long firm strokes. Repeat several times. Move your hands to the back of each leg in turn and press the flesh firmly, lifting it and pushing against the skin. Work the flesh back and forwards, taking care not to "burn" it. Afterwards relax, listen to some music and drink a glass of fresh juice or a cup of herbal tea.

6.00pm Evening meal. Prepare a large plate of lightly steamed vegetables and season it with fresh herbs, nuts, and seeds. Again, eat it slowly and be aware of each mouthful as you chew it. Remember, take time for it to digest.

7.00pm Visualization. Sit in a quiet room and focus all your thoughts on pleasing, positive images. Whenever random thoughts intervene, brush them aside and focus on the image in your mind's eye.

8.00pm Have a pleasant aromatherapy bath. Make sure the bathroom is warm and relaxing. Light the room with candles and play some of your favorite music. As you lie luxuriating in the warmth and listening to the music, begin taking deep breaths and, as you slowly exhale, feel the tensions ebbing away. After your bath, dry yourself, put on your nightwear and relax with a soothing cup of herbal tea.

Don't forget: As you complete each activity, tick it off on your chart. Before you go to sleep, remember to record in your diary how you felt, writing down both the good and the bad points.

Remainder of the week

For the remainder of week you should follow the same basic routine but choose some different foods, and experiment with different recipes. On day 3 exfoliate the skin and on day 5 take an Epsom salts bath. By day 6 you may start to feel a little bored, so make it more exciting by adding in extra little treats – have a manicure, give yourself a facial, watch a film one afternoon. Introducing subtle changes into the program will help to maintain your interest.

End of the first week
- You will feel more alert
- Your skin will have taken on a better color
- There may be spots on your back but these are the result of the toxins leaving your body
- You should feel fitter and look leaner because of the exercise

Measurements chart

The detox program is not a weight-loss diet, but as you change your routine and reform your eating habits, you will find that you are not only looking good and feeling better, but you will have more energy and will have toned up those muscles too! You can record your measurements each week using this simple chart.

	Week 1	Week 2	Week 3	Week 4
Date				
Weight				
Bust				
Waist				
Hips				

Detox Days 8–14

You will have established a routine by now and perhaps made some changes to the overall schedule. So are you ready for week two?

7.00am Glass of hot water and lemon or lime juice. Skin brush, then a quick shower.

8.00am Breakfast – a large bowl of fresh fruit salad.

9.00am Have a facial sauna.

11.00am Visualization.

1.00pm Lunch – a nice, crunchy salad.

2.30pm Go for a swim. It will be time for some relaxation when you return home.

3.15pm Relaxation. Have a glass of herbal tea and an orange afterward.

6.00pm Evening meal – stir-fried vegetables.

8.00pm Take an oatmeal bath (see box). Afterwards massage your feet with lots of moisturizer, then put on a pair of cotton socks. The perspiration from your feet will blend with the cream and leave your skin silky soft.

Don't forget: As you complete each activity, tick it off on your chart. Before you go to sleep, remember to write up your diary.

Remainder of the week

Keep up with the routine, even if you don't feel like it on some days. If you really feel down in the dumps, do something positive – go along to your local gym for a workout, and don't forget that a good dose of active housework is just as beneficial as a 35-minute swim in the pool. You may well be tempted to weigh yourself at this stage. If you have followed the program correctly, you will probably have lost some weight.

Oatmeal bath

While the body is detoxing, the skin can sometimes become rather irritated. To alleviate this, try taking an oatmeal bath; it is very calming and soothing • Tie 1lb of uncooked oatmeal in an old pantyhose and hang it under the hot water faucet when running your bath • As the water flows through the oats, they will release their calming agents • Drop the oatmeal pantyhose into the water or use it as a sponge • Relax for about 20 minutes, long enough to allow the chemicals from the oats to infiltrate the skin • Then gently pat skin dry with a towel.

Changes that you should feel:
- Not so tired in the evening
- More alert and refreshed when you waken in the morning
- Your skin will look a lot better and any spots will probably have vanished
- You will be feeling much fitter and your body will look toned
- Your energy levels will be higher

Detox Days 15–21

You are now embarking on the second half of your detox program. It probably hasn't been easy to get this far, but there is no turning back now.

You have come a long way and your body will be reaping the rewards of your endeavors.

7.00am Glass of hot water and lemon/lime juice. Skin brush, then a quick shower.
8.00am Breakfast – mix dried apricot seeds together and sprinkle them over the top of yogurt.
9.00am Give yourself a massage using some of your favourite aromatherapy essential oils.
11.00am Do some strenuous housework, vacuuming the carpets or washing the windows. The secret is to do it in half the time that you would normally take. So if a job usually takes you two hours, make sure that this time it only takes you one hour.
1.00pm Lunch – perhaps try some carrot soup.
2.00pm Visualization. At the end of the session, give yourself a facial sauna.
3.15pm Relaxation or try some yoga. Curl up with a book.
6.00pm Evening meal – you might choose some fish and a salad.
8.00pm Bath, then treat yourself to a manicure and pedicure.

Don't forget: As you complete each activity, tick it off on your chart. Before you go to sleep, remember to write up your diary.

Remainder of the week
Keep changing the foods you eat, the exercises you do and remember to keep including those little treats.

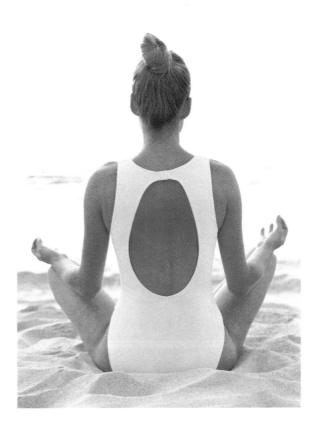

Changes that you should feel:
- Feeling totally refreshed and energetic
- Your skin should be smooth and unblemished with no dry patches
- You should have lost some weight
- Your body will feel and look much firmer
- The muscles at the tops of your arms and legs will be more defined
- You will feel on a high knowing that your body is now cleansed and working at its optimum level

Detox Days 22–28

Finally you are on the last lap. By now you have probably established a great routine of your own which may seem like second nature to you.

Now is not the time to give up or to falter. Keep going – only seven days to the finish!

7.00am Glass of hot water and lemon/lime juice. Skin brush, then a quick shower.

8.00am Breakfast – try a bowl of fresh fruit salad (you might want to prepare it the night before).

9.00am Breathing exercises. Give yourself a facial scrub.

11.00am Do some trampolining if you have one, or take yourself along to the local gym and enjoy a stimulating workout.

1.00pm Lunch – treat yourself to a tasty potato salad with fennel.

2.00pm Total relaxation.

3.15pm Visualization.

6.00pm Evening meal – a selection of roast vegetables might be nice.

8.00pm Take an Epsom salts bath.

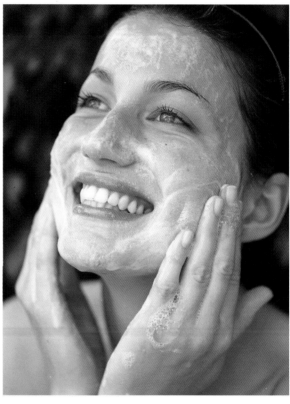

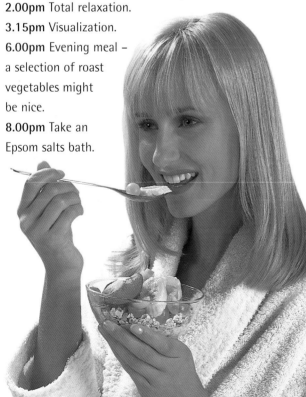

The new you is revealed!

- Your skin will look better than it has for years
- Exercise will have become an integral part of your life
- Your body will look and feel in great shape
- You will feel on a total high – and so you should
- This is the healthiest you will have felt for years

Now is the time to weigh yourself and record your measurements in the chart on page 27. Look back at your original measurements to see how well you have done.

Activity Record Chart

Record your activities every day using this table

DAILY ACTIVITIES	1	2	3	4	5	6	7	8	9	10	11	12	13	14	15	16	17	18	19	20	21	22	23	24	25	26	27	28
Glass of hot water and lemon or lime juice																												
Shower/bath																												
Skin brushing																												
Moisturizing																												
Breakfast																												
Lunch																												
Dinner																												
3 pints water																												
Fruit																												
Goat's/sheep's milk																												
Goat's/sheep's cheese																												
Brown rice																												
Salad																												
Nuts																												
10 mins relaxation																												
5 mins breathing																												
5 mins visualization																												
Pampering																												
Exfoliate every three days																												
Laugh																												
Massage																												
Epsom salts bath 6 times during program																												

Congratulations!

You've done it! You've successfully completed the 28-day detox program. You will probably feel healthier than you have done for ages and you can be very proud of yourself.

Not only have you succeeded in cleansing your body of toxins, but in so doing you have emerged a fitter, happier, and more confident person. But make sure, as you ride this wave of euphoria, that you don't slide back. You've come so far in the last 28 days that you don't want to risk losing all the hard-won gains.

Old habits are difficult to break, but during those dark moments when you felt that you couldn't continue, you didn't let those doubts undermine your determination. And now you have achieved this peak of good health, make sure that you hold on to it.

After all, you are the only person who can ensure that you do!

Try to make these recommendations part of your everyday life:
- Drink hot water and lemon/lime juice first thing in the morning
- Drink 3 pints of water every day
- Take the liver tonics daily – a snack of some black grapes plus a cup of fennel tea isn't hard to remember
- Take two kidney tonics each day – try adding a teaspoon of honey to your lemon juice and adding a cranberry supplement at breakfast time
- Eat three sensible meals a day

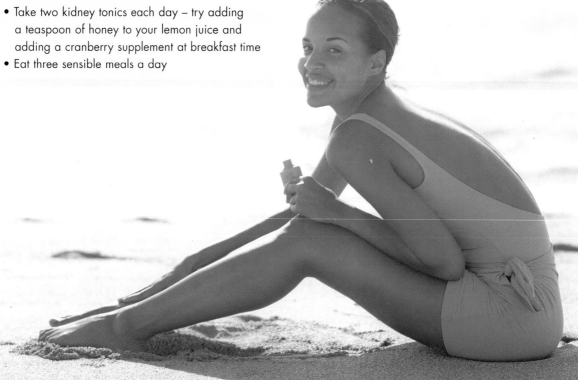